I0698221

Simple Exercises For Osteoporosis

Simple Exercises For Osteoporosis

Approaches to Building Resilient Bones and Preventing Fractures

Victor Asher

ISBN-13: 9798394290572

DEDICTAION

This book is dedicated to God Almighty for His grace and wisdom, my family members, my wonderful readers who will find this book relevant to them and all those who have loved, supported, and encouraged me throughout my journey. Without your unwavering belief in me, I would not be where I am today. I dedicate this book to those struggling with bone issues, and I desire this helps you out and keep   you   all   fit.

CONTENTS

ACKNOWLEDGMENT

I would like to express my sincere gratitude to God for the enablement and wisdom that saw me through the creation of this book. To my editor and publisher, thank you for your invaluable guidance and support in shaping this manuscript into its final form. To the individuals who generously shared their time and expertise, thank you for enriching this project with your insights. To my family members who have been a source of motivation and strength to me, their encouragements and support. I also extend this gratitude to my friends and loved ones, thank you for your unwavering love and support throughout the process. My sincere gratitude goes to my readers, thank you for taking the time to engage with this work. It is my hope that it will inspire and provoke thought in equal measure. You all are wonderful and I really appreciate every one of you.

Introduction

Osteoporosis is a medical condition characterized by the progressive loss of bone density and strength, resulting in increased risk of fractures. The word "osteoporosis" comes from the Greek words for "porous bones," reflecting the fact that bones affected by this condition become fragile and more likely to break, even with minor trauma.

Osteoporosis is most commonly associated with aging, but it can also occur due to hormonal changes, nutritional deficiencies, and certain medical conditions or medications. Treatment for osteoporosis typically involves a combination of lifestyle modifications, such as exercise and a healthy diet, as well as medications to help slow or reverse bone loss.

Some common medications used to treat osteoporosis include bisphosphonates, which help to slow down bone breakdown and reduce the risk of fractures, and selective estrogen receptor modulators (SERMs), which can help to increase bone density and reduce fracture risk in postmenopausal women. Other medications that may be used to treat osteoporosis include calcitonin, teriparatide, and denosumab.

It is important for individuals at risk of osteoporosis to take steps to prevent the condition before it develops. This includes ensuring adequate intake of calcium and vitamin D, engaging in regular weight-bearing exercise, avoiding smoking and excessive alcohol consumption, and getting regular bone density testing. For individuals who have already been diagnosed with osteoporosis, ongoing treatment and monitoring is necessary to help prevent fractures and maintain bone health.

Chapter One

What Causes Osteoporosis?

Osteoporosis is a bone disease that happens when bone mass and mineral density diminish or when there are changes to the way that bones are built and how strong they are. The risk of fractures (broken bones) may rise as a result of a reduction in bone strength. There are several factors that can contribute to the development of osteoporosis.

1. Age

One of the most significant risk factors for osteoporosis is age. As people age, their bones become less dense and lose calcium, making them weaker and more susceptible to fractures. This process typically begins in women around the time of menopause, when estrogen levels decline, and bone loss accelerates.

2. Gender

Women are more likely than men to develop osteoporosis, primarily due to the rapid decline in estrogen levels that occurs after menopause. Estrogen plays an essential role in maintaining bone density, and the loss of estrogen after menopause can lead to accelerated bone loss.

3. Genetics

Genetics also play a role in the development of osteoporosis. Individuals with a family history of the condition are at increased risk, as are those with certain genetic disorders that affect bone metabolism, such as osteogenesis imperfecta.

4. Lifestyle factors

Certain lifestyle factors can also contribute to the development of osteoporosis.

These include:

- Low calcium and vitamin D intake

Calcium and vitamin D are essential for strong bones, and low intake of these nutrients can increase the risk of osteoporosis.

- Lack of physical activity

Regular exercise helps to strengthen bones and prevent bone loss. Individuals who are sedentary are at increased risk of osteoporosis.

- Smoking

Smoking can lead to decreased bone density, as it impairs the body's ability to absorb calcium and reduces estrogen levels.

- Excessive alcohol consumption

Heavy alcohol consumption can increase the risk of osteoporosis, as it can interfere with the body's ability to absorb calcium and affect hormone levels.

5. Medical conditions

Certain medical conditions can also increase the risk of osteoporosis.

These include:

- Hormonal disorders

Conditions that affect hormone levels, such as hyperthyroidism or Cushing's syndrome, can lead to bone loss.

Chronic kidney disease

Individuals with chronic kidney disease are at increased risk of osteoporosis due to alterations in calcium and phosphorus metabolism.

- Rheumatoid arthritis

Chronic inflammation associated with rheumatoid arthritis can lead to bone loss.

- Cancer and its treatments

Certain types of cancer, as well as treatments such as chemotherapy and hormone therapy, can increase the risk of osteoporosis.

6. Medications:

Certain medications can also increase the risk of osteoporosis.

These include:

- Glucocorticoids

These medications, commonly used to treat conditions such as asthma and rheumatoid arthritis, can lead to bone loss with long-term use.

- Some anticonvulsants

These medications can interfere with the body's ability to absorb calcium, leading to bone loss.

- Some cancer treatments

Certain cancer treatments, such as aromatase inhibitors and gonadotropin-releasing hormone agonists, can increase the risk of osteoporosis.

In summary, osteoporosis is a multifactorial condition with several risk factors. While some of these risk factors, such as age and genetics, are beyond an individual's control, there are lifestyle modifications that can help reduce the risk of osteoporosis, such as regular exercise, a balanced diet rich in calcium and vitamin D, and avoidance of smoking and excessive alcohol consumption.

Additionally, early detection and treatment of underlying medical conditions that contribute to bone loss can help prevent or slow the progression of osteoporosis. Healthcare providers play a critical role in identifying individuals at risk for osteoporosis and recommending appropriate interventions to reduce the risk of fractures and other complications.

Chapter Two

Risk Factors and Diagnosis of Osteoporosis

Osteoporosis is a condition characterized by weakened bones that are more prone to fractures. It is often called the "silent disease" because there are usually no symptoms until a fracture occurs. Therefore, diagnosis of osteoporosis typically involves assessing the risk factors, conducting bone mineral density (BMD) tests, and evaluating for fractures.

Risk Factors

The risk factors for osteoporosis include advanced age, female sex, low body weight, a family history of osteoporosis, low calcium and vitamin D intake, lack of physical activity, smoking, excessive alcohol consumption, and certain medical conditions such as hyperthyroidism, chronic kidney disease, and rheumatoid arthritis. Healthcare providers will typically ask about these factors during the evaluation.

Diagnosis of Osteoporosis

There are several methods used to diagnose osteoporosis, and these include:

1. Bone mineral density (BMD) testing

This is the most common method used to diagnose osteoporosis. BMD testing uses a special X-ray machine called a dual-energy X-ray absorptiometry (DXA) scanner to measure bone density at various points in the body, such as the spine, hips, and wrists.

BMD testing is considered the gold standard for the diagnosis of osteoporosis. It can detect early bone loss before a fracture occurs and measure changes in bone density over time.

The results of BMD testing are reported as a T-score, which compares an individual's bone density to that of a healthy young adult of the same gender. A T-score of -2.5 or lower indicates osteoporosis, while a T-score between -1.0 and -2.5 indicates osteopenia, a condition of low bone density that may lead to osteoporosis if left untreated.

2. Blood tests

Blood tests can be useful in diagnosing osteoporosis as it can be used to measure levels of certain hormones and minerals that are important for bone health, such as calcium, vitamin D, and parathyroid hormone. In addition to measuring calcium, vitamin D, and parathyroid hormone levels, blood tests can also be used to measure levels of bone-specific proteins, such as alkaline phosphatase and osteocalcin, which can indicate bone turnover and help assess fracture risk.

Blood tests can also help identify underlying medical conditions that may contribute to osteoporosis, such as hyperthyroidism or chronic kidney disease.

3. Imaging tests

Other imaging tests, such as CT scans or MRIs, may be used to look for signs of osteoporosis, such as fractures or changes in bone structure.

While CT scans and MRIs are not typically used as the primary means of diagnosing osteoporosis, they can be helpful in certain situations. For example, if a patient has a fracture that is suspected to be related to osteoporosis, a CT scan or MRI may be ordered to confirm the diagnosis and assess the severity of the fracture.

In addition, some newer imaging techniques may be used to evaluate bone quality and strength, which can provide additional information about a patient's risk for fractures. For example, trabecular bone score (TBS) is a method of analyzing the structure of the trabecular bone (the spongy interior of bones) using DXA scans. TBS can help to identify patients who are at increased risk of fractures, even if their BMD is not significantly low.

Another imaging technique that may be used in certain cases is quantitative computed tomography (QCT), which is a type of CT scan that can provide more detailed information about bone density and strength than traditional DXA scans. QCT may be used in patients who have metal implants or other factors that make DXA testing difficult or unreliable.

4. Fracture risk assessment

Doctors may use a tool called FRAX (Fracture Risk Assessment) to estimate an individual's risk of experiencing a fracture in the next 10 years based on factors such as age, gender, and medical history.

FRAX is a tool that takes into account several clinical risk factors, including age, sex, weight, height, previous fractures, family history of hip fractures, smoking status, alcohol intake, and use of glucocorticoids, as well as the results of BMD testing, to estimate the 10-year probability of a major osteoporotic fracture (including clinical spine, hip, forearm, and shoulder fractures) and the 10-year probability of a hip fracture. FRAX can help guide decisions about whether to start treatment for osteoporosis and what type of treatment to use.

It's important to note that osteoporosis is often referred to as a "silent disease" because it can progress for many years without causing any symptoms. Therefore, early detection through screening and testing is crucial in the prevention and management of the condition.

In addition to these tests, healthcare providers may also perform blood tests to assess for medical conditions that may contribute to osteoporosis, such as hyperthyroidism or kidney disease. Imaging studies such as X-rays or CT scans may also be used to evaluate for fractures or other bone abnormalities.

Overall, diagnosis of osteoporosis involves assessing risk factors, conducting BMD tests, and evaluating for fractures. It is important to diagnose and treat osteoporosis early to prevent fractures and reduce the risk of complications. Healthcare providers play a critical role in diagnosing and managing osteoporosis, and individuals who are at risk or have concerns should speak with their healthcare provider to determine the appropriate course of action.

Chapter Three

Why You Need Exercise for Osteoporosis

Regular exercise is crucial for maintaining healthy bones, especially for individuals with osteoporosis. When you engage in physical activity, it places a healthy amount of stress on your bones, which stimulates bone growth and helps maintain bone density. As a result, regular exercise can help prevent or slow down the progression of osteoporosis, reduce the risk of falls and fractures, and improve overall bone health and strength.

One of the main reasons exercise is important for osteoporosis is because it helps to increase bone density. Bone density refers to the amount of minerals, such as calcium and phosphorus that are present in your bones. The greater the bone density, the stronger and more resistant the bone is to fractures.

When you engage in weight-bearing exercises, such as walking, jogging, dancing, or lifting weights, it places stress on your bones. This stress stimulates the cells in your bones to build more bone tissue, which can increase bone density over time.

Exercise can also help to improve bone quality. Bones are made up of living tissue that constantly undergoes a process called remodeling. During remodeling, old bone tissue is broken down and replaced with new bone tissue. When you engage in physical activity, it triggers the remodeling process and helps to create stronger, more durable bone tissue.

Another important benefit of exercise for osteoporosis is that it can help to reduce the risk of falls and fractures. Falls are a major concern for individuals with osteoporosis because their bones are more fragile and susceptible to fracture. Regular exercise can help to improve balance, coordination, and flexibility, all of which are important factors in preventing falls. Additionally, exercise can help to strengthen the muscles around your bones, which can help to absorb the impact of a fall and reduce the risk of fractures.

Finally, exercise can help to improve overall health and well-being, which is important for individuals with osteoporosis who may be at a higher risk for other health problems. Exercise can help to improve cardiovascular health, lower blood pressure, improve mood and mental health, and reduce the risk of chronic diseases such as diabetes and heart disease.

In conclusion, exercise is an essential component of managing osteoporosis. It can help to increase bone density, improve bone quality, reduce the risk of falls and fractures, and improve overall health and well-being. If you have osteoporosis, it is important to work with your healthcare provider to develop an exercise plan that is safe and effective for your individual needs and abilities.

By incorporating regular exercise into your lifestyle, you can help to maintain healthy bones and reduce the risk of fractures and other complications associated with osteoporosis.

How Exercise Helps Build Strong Bones

Exercise plays a crucial role in building strong bones by stimulating the process of bone remodeling. Bone remodeling is a continuous process in which old bone tissue is broken down and replaced with new bone tissue. During this process, specialized cells called osteoblasts are responsible for building new bone tissue, while another type of cell called osteoclasts break down old bone tissue. When the rate of bone breakdown is higher than the rate of bone formation, it can lead to a loss of bone density and strength, which is a characteristic of osteoporosis.

Engaging in regular exercise can help to stimulate bone remodeling by placing stress on the bones. Specifically, weight-bearing exercises, such as walking, running, jumping, and strength training, can help to create small micro-fractures in the bones. These micro-fractures signal the body to increase the production of osteoblasts and accelerate the process of bone remodeling.

In addition to stimulating the process of bone remodeling, exercise also helps to increase bone density by promoting the absorption of calcium and other minerals into the bones. Calcium is an essential mineral that is required for bone growth and maintenance. When you engage in weight-bearing exercises, the muscles pull on the bones, which causes the bones to flex slightly. This flexing action creates small electrical currents in the bones, which can help to stimulate the absorption of calcium and other minerals into the bone tissue.

Another way that exercise helps to build strong bones is by promoting the production of hormones that are important for bone health. For example, exercise can help to increase the production of growth hormone and testosterone, both of which are important for bone growth and maintenance. Exercise can also help to increase the production of estrogen in women, which is important for maintaining bone density and strength.

It is important to note that not all types of exercise are equally effective for building strong bones. Weight-bearing exercises, which place stress on the bones, are the most effective for stimulating bone growth and maintenance. Examples of weight-bearing exercises include walking, jogging, dancing, and strength training. Non-weight-bearing exercises, such as swimming and cycling, are less effective for building bone density because they do not place stress on the bones.

Finally, regular exercise is an important component of building strong bones and maintaining bone density and strength. Weight-bearing exercises are the most effective for stimulating the process of bone remodeling and promoting the absorption of calcium and other minerals into the bones. By incorporating regular exercise into your lifestyle, you can help to maintain healthy bones and reduce the risk of fractures and other complications associated with osteoporosis.

Chapter Four

Bone Remodeling Process

Bone remodeling is a continuous process that occurs throughout our lives, in which old bone tissue is removed and new bone tissue is formed. This process is essential for maintaining healthy bone density and strength, and for repairing bone tissue after injury.

The process of bone remodeling involves two main types of cells: osteoclasts and osteoblasts. Osteoclasts are cells that are responsible for breaking down old bone tissue. They secrete enzymes and acids that dissolve the minerals in the bone, and then digest the collagen fibers that make up the bone matrix. The result is the formation of small cavities, or resorption pits, on the bone surface.

After the old bone tissue has been removed, osteoblasts move in to form new bone tissue. Osteoblasts are cells that produce the proteins and minerals that make up the bone matrix. They secrete collagen, which forms the scaffolding for the new bone tissue, and they also secrete proteins that help to mineralize the bone, such as calcium and phosphate. Over time, the new bone tissue becomes mineralized and hard, and it forms a new layer on top of the existing bone.

The process of bone remodeling is regulated by a complex network of hormones, growth factors, and signaling molecules. These factors help to control the balance between bone resorption and bone formation, and they also help to coordinate the activity of osteoclasts and osteoblasts.

One of the most important factors that regulate bone remodeling is mechanical stress. When bones are subjected to stress, such as during weight-bearing exercise, the cells in the bone tissue sense the stress and respond by increasing bone formation. This is why weight-bearing exercise is so important for building strong bones and maintaining bone density and strength.

Other factors that can affect bone remodeling include nutritional status, hormonal changes, and certain medical conditions. For example, a diet that is low in calcium and vitamin D can impair bone formation, while hormonal changes associated with menopause can increase bone resorption and lead to bone loss.

In summary, bone remodeling is a continuous process that is essential for maintaining healthy bones. The process involves the coordinated activity of osteoclasts and osteoblasts, and it is regulated by a complex network of hormones and signaling molecules. By engaging in weight-bearing exercise and maintaining a healthy diet, we can help to promote bone remodeling and maintain healthy bone density and strength.

Phases of Bone Remodeling

The process of bone remodeling can be divided into several distinct phases, each with its own unique characteristics and cellular events. These phases include:

1. Activation

The first phase of bone remodeling is activation. During this phase, osteoclasts are recruited to the site of the bone that needs to be remodeled. Osteoclasts are specialized cells that break down and resorb old bone tissue, and they are responsible for removing damaged or old bone tissue during the remodeling process. This recruitment is controlled by a variety of signaling molecules, including cytokines, growth factors, and hormones, which are released by other cells in the bone microenvironment.

Once the osteoclasts have been recruited, they attach to the surface of the bone tissue and begin to resorb or break down the old bone tissue. This process involves the secretion of enzymes and acid, which dissolve the mineralized bone tissue and break down the collagen matrix of the bone. The osteoclasts create small cavities or pits on the bone surface, which will later be filled in by new bone tissue.

The activation phase is an important step in the bone remodeling process, as it allows the body to selectively target and remove damaged or old bone tissue, and replace it with new tissue. This process helps to maintain bone density and strength, and is essential for repairing bone damage and adapting to changes in mechanical loading.

However, excessive activation of osteoclasts can lead to bone loss and osteoporosis, while insufficient activation can lead to bone mineralization disorders such as osteopetrosis. Therefore, it is important to maintain a balance between bone resorption and formation during the bone remodeling process, which can be achieved through a variety of factors such as exercise, nutrition, and hormone regulation.

2. Resorption

The second phase of bone remodeling is resorption and it is initiated by the activation of osteoclasts. During this phase, osteoclasts resorb or break down the old bone tissue by dissolving the mineralized bone tissue and breaking down the collagen matrix of the bone. This process creates small cavities or pits on the bone surface, which will later be filled in by new bone tissue.

The process of resorption involves the secretion of enzymes and acid, which dissolve the mineralized bone tissue, including hydrochloric acid, lysosomal enzymes, and proteases. The osteoclasts attach to the bone surface through integrin receptors and form a sealing zone, creating a microenvironment for acidification and enzymatic digestion of the bone tissue.

As the osteoclasts dissolve the mineralized bone tissue, they create small cavities or pits on the bone surface, which are called resorption pits or Howship's lacunae. These pits allow the osteoclasts to gain access to the deeper layers of the bone tissue and break down the collagen matrix of the bone.

The resorption phase is an important step in the bone remodeling process, as it allows the body to selectively remove damaged or old bone tissue and replace it with new tissue. However, excessive resorption can lead to bone loss and osteoporosis, while insufficient resorption can lead to abnormal bone growth and mineralization disorders such as osteopetrosis.

The balance between resorption and formation is regulated by a variety of factors, including hormones such as parathyroid hormone and calcitonin, growth factors, and cytokines. This balance is essential for maintaining healthy bone density and strength and adapting to changes in mechanical loading. Exercise, nutrition, and hormone regulation can all play important roles in promoting healthy bone remodeling and preventing bone loss and other bone-related disorders.

3. Reversal

After the bone tissue has been resorbed, the remodeling process enters the reversal phase. During this phase, the activity of the osteoclasts decreases, and the bone tissue begins to undergo repair and rebuilding.

The reversal phase is a critical transition point in the bone remodeling process, as it marks the transition from bone resorption to bone formation. During this phase, a group of cells called osteoblasts are recruited to the resorption pits created by the osteoclasts. Osteoblasts are responsible for synthesizing and depositing new bone tissue, including the collagen matrix and mineralized bone tissue.

The recruitment of osteoblasts to the site of bone remodeling is regulated by a variety of signaling molecules, including growth factors and cytokines. Once they are recruited, the osteoblasts begin to synthesize and deposit new bone tissue on the resorption pit surface, creating a new layer of bone tissue.

The reversal phase is a critical step in the bone remodeling process, as it allows the body to repair and rebuild the damaged or old bone tissue that was removed during the resorption phase. This process helps to maintain bone density and strength, and is essential for repairing bone damage and adapting to changes in mechanical loading.

However, if the balance between resorption and formation is disrupted, bone density and strength can be compromised, leading to bone loss and osteoporosis. Therefore, it is important to maintain a healthy balance between resorption and formation through a variety of factors, including exercise, nutrition, and hormone regulation.

4. Formation

The fourth phase of bone remodeling is formation. During this phase, osteoblasts move in and begin to produce new bone tissue to replace the old tissue that was resorbed. Osteoblasts produce a collagen matrix that becomes mineralized with calcium and other minerals, creating new bone tissue.

As we mentioned earlier, osteoblasts are specialized cells that synthesize and deposit new bone tissue, including the collagen matrix and mineralized bone tissue. During the formation phase, the osteoblasts begin to lay down a new collagen matrix on the surface of the resorption pit. The collagen matrix then becomes mineralized with calcium and other minerals, creating new bone tissue.

The process of bone formation is regulated by a variety of signaling molecules, including growth factors and hormones. These molecules help to stimulate the activity of the osteoblasts and promote the deposition of new bone tissue.

The rate of bone formation can vary depending on a variety of factors, including age, hormonal status, and mechanical loading. In general, bone formation tends to be most active during childhood and adolescence, when bones are growing and developing. As we age, the rate of bone formation tends to slow down, which can contribute to the development of osteoporosis.

However, regular exercise can help to stimulate bone formation and promote the deposition of new bone tissue. Weight-bearing and resistance exercises, in particular, have been shown to be effective at stimulating bone formation and increasing bone density, which can help to reduce the risk of osteoporosis and fractures.

Overall, the formation phase of bone remodeling is essential for maintaining bone health and strength. By promoting the deposition of new bone tissue, the body is able to repair and rebuild bone tissue that has been damaged or lost, and maintain bone density and strength over time.

5. Mineralization

The final phase of bone remodeling is mineralization, also known as the maturation or ossification phase. During this phase, the newly formed bone tissue undergoes a process of mineralization, in which the bone matrix becomes infiltrated with minerals such as calcium, phosphate, and hydroxyl ions. This process gives the bone tissue its characteristic hardness and strength, and ultimately allows it to function effectively in supporting the body and protecting internal organs.

The process of mineralization is tightly regulated by a variety of hormones and signaling molecules, including vitamin D, parathyroid hormone, and calcitonin. These molecules help to maintain the proper balance of calcium and other minerals in the body, and ensure that bone tissue is mineralized to the appropriate degree.

As the mineralization process continues, the newly formed bone tissue gradually replaces the old bone tissue that was resorbed during the earlier phases of bone remodeling. Over time, this process helps to maintain the strength and integrity of the bone tissue, and ensures that it is able to withstand the stresses and strains of everyday movement and activity.

It is important to note that mineralization is a dynamic process that continues throughout life, and can be influenced by a variety of factors. For example, factors such as age, hormonal status, and nutritional status can all impact the rate and extent of bone mineralization. In addition, lifestyle factors such as exercise and smoking can also have a significant impact on bone health and mineralization.

Regular weight-bearing and resistance exercise has been shown to be particularly effective at promoting bone mineralization and increasing bone density. By stimulating the activity of osteoblasts and promoting the deposition of new bone tissue, exercise helps to maintain the strength and integrity of the bone tissue, and reduces the risk of fractures and other bone-related injuries.

In summary, the final phase of bone remodeling is mineralization, in which newly formed bone tissue becomes mineralized with calcium and other minerals, giving it its characteristic hardness and strength. This process is essential for maintaining the strength and integrity of the bone tissue, and can be influenced by a variety of factors, including age, hormonal status, nutritional status, and lifestyle factors such as exercise.

The Role of Exercise in Bone Remodeling

The role of exercise in bone remodeling is essential for maintaining bone health and preventing bone-related injuries. Exercise can stimulate the activity of osteoblasts, promoting the formation of new bone tissue, while also reducing the activity of osteoclasts, preventing excessive bone resorption. Regular exercise, particularly weight-bearing and resistance exercises, can also improve overall bone density, making the bones stronger and more resistant to fractures. By incorporating exercise into their daily routine, individuals can help to promote bone remodeling and maintain strong, healthy bones throughout their lives.

The role of exercise in bone remodeling includes:

1. Stimulating osteoblast activity

Osteoblasts are bone cells that are responsible for producing new bone tissue. Exercise can stimulate osteoblasts to produce new bone tissue, which can increase bone density and strength.

Exercise, particularly weight-bearing and resistance exercises, can stimulate the activity of osteoblasts and promote the production of new bone tissue. When bones are subjected to mechanical loading, such as during weight-bearing exercise, osteoblasts become activated and begin to produce new bone tissue. This process can help to increase bone density and improve bone strength, reducing the risk of fractures in individuals with osteoporosis.

2. Increasing mechanical stress on bones

Weight-bearing and resistance exercises create stress on bones, which stimulates bone remodeling and helps to maintain or improve bone density and strength.

When bones experience mechanical stress, such as during weight-bearing and resistance exercises, it triggers the osteoblasts to produce more bone tissue in order to adapt to the increased demand. This process is called "bone modeling" and it leads to stronger and denser bones.

The bone tissue that is produced in response to mechanical stress is oriented along the lines of the stress, which further enhances the strength and resilience of the bone.

Therefore, exercises that place mechanical stress on bones, such as weight-bearing exercises like walking, jogging, and stair climbing, as well as resistance exercises like weight lifting and bodyweight exercises, can help to increase bone density and improve bone strength.

3. Enhancing calcium uptake

Exercise can enhance the uptake of calcium in bones, which is essential for bone mineralization and strengthening.

Adequate calcium intake is indeed essential for maintaining healthy bones, and exercise can enhance calcium uptake and utilization in the bones, but it cannot replace the need for adequate calcium intake. The National Osteoporosis Foundation recommends that adults aged 50 and older consume 1,200 mg of calcium per day, either through diet or supplements, along with vitamin D, which is necessary for calcium absorption.

In addition to weight-bearing exercises, resistance training has also been shown to improve calcium metabolism in the body. When the muscles contract during resistance exercises, they release calcium ions into the bloodstream, which can be taken up by the bones for mineralization. This process can help to increase overall calcium utilization in the body and improve bone health.

It's important to note that too much exercise or excessive training can have negative effects on bone health. Overtraining and excessive physical activity can lead to hormonal imbalances, such as decreased estrogen levels in women, which can increase the risk of osteoporosis. Therefore, it's essential to engage in regular exercise at an appropriate intensity and duration to maximize the benefits for bone health. Consulting with a healthcare professional or a certified exercise specialist can help individuals develop safe and effective exercise programs for maintaining and improving bone health.

4. Reducing bone resorption

Exercise can help to reduce bone resorption by decreasing the activity of osteoclasts (the cells responsible for breaking down old bone tissue, which can help to slow down bone loss). This is important because excessive bone resorption can lead to bone loss and weaken the bones, increasing the risk of fractures.

Studies have shown that exercise, particularly weight-bearing and resistance exercises, can help to reduce bone resorption by inhibiting the activity of osteoclasts. These exercises create mechanical stress on the bones, which can signal the body to decrease the activity of osteoclasts and reduce bone resorption. Additionally, certain types of exercise, such as high-impact exercises, have been shown to stimulate the production of osteoprotegerin, a protein that helps to regulate bone resorption.

Reducing bone resorption is an important aspect of maintaining healthy bones, especially for individuals with osteoporosis. By decreasing the activity of osteoclasts, exercise can help to slow down bone loss and preserve bone density, ultimately reducing the risk of fractures.

5. Improving balance and coordination

Exercise that focuses on balance and coordination, such as yoga or tai chi, can help to reduce the risk of falls and fractures, which are a common complication of osteoporosis.

Falls and fractures are a significant concern for individuals with osteoporosis, as weakened bones are more prone to breaking even from a minor fall. Improving balance and coordination can help individuals maintain their stability and avoid falls.

Exercise programs that incorporate specific balance and coordination exercises, such as yoga or tai chi, can help to improve proprioception (awareness of the body's position and movement) and neuromuscular control, which can reduce the risk of falls and fractures.

These exercises often involve slow, controlled movements, and can be modified to meet individual needs and abilities.

6. Boosting hormone production

Exercise can increase the production of hormones that are essential for bone health, such as growth hormone, testosterone, and estrogen.

Exercise can stimulate the production of hormones that are essential for bone health. Growth hormone is known to stimulate bone growth and increase bone density, while testosterone is important for maintaining muscle mass and bone strength in men. In women, estrogen is important for maintaining bone density, and exercise can help to increase estrogen production.

However, it is important to note that the effects of exercise on hormone production may vary depending on factors such as age, sex, and the type and intensity of exercise.

7. Increasing blood flow

Exercise increases blood flow to bones, which can help to deliver essential nutrients and minerals needed for bone remodeling and strengthening.

Exercise can help to increase blood flow to the bones, this increased blood flow can also help to remove waste products and promote healing. In addition, exercise can improve overall circulation in the body, which can benefit the bones and other organs.

Overall, exercise plays a critical role in bone remodeling by promoting bone formation, reducing bone resorption, and improving bone density and strength. Regular exercise is essential for maintaining good bone health and reducing the risk of osteoporosis and   fractures.

Chapter Five

Exercises that Promote Bone Health

There are several types of exercises that promote bone health and can be beneficial for individuals with osteoporosis. These include:

1. Weight-bearing exercises

Weight-bearing exercises involve activities where the feet and legs support the body's weight. Examples include walking, jogging, dancing, stair climbing, and hiking. These exercises place stress on the bones, which can stimulate bone remodeling and increase bone density.

Weight-bearing exercises are considered one of the best types of exercise for promoting bone health and reducing the risk of osteoporosis. These exercises can be performed in a variety of ways and can be adapted to suit different fitness levels and abilities.

- **Walking**

Walking is one of the simplest and most accessible weight-bearing exercises. It can be performed indoors or outdoors and requires no special equipment. Walking at a brisk pace for at least 30 minutes a day can help to stimulate bone remodeling and increase bone density.

- **Jogging and running**

They are higher-impact weight-bearing exercises that can be more challenging but also more effective at stimulating bone remodeling. These exercises involve a greater degree of impact and stress on the bones and can help to increase bone density in the legs and hips.

- **Dancing**

Dancing is another fun and effective weight-bearing exercise that can help to improve bone health. Dancing involves a variety of movements and steps that can help to stimulate bone remodeling and increase bone density.

- **Stair climbing**

Stair climbing is a weight-bearing exercise that can be performed indoors or outdoors. It involves climbing up and down stairs or using a stair-stepping machine. This exercise can help to strengthen the bones in the legs and hips and improve overall cardiovascular health.

- **Hiking**

Hiking is a weight-bearing exercise that can be performed outdoors in natural settings such as mountains, forests, and parks. Hiking involves walking over uneven terrain and up and down hills, which can provide a challenging workout for the bones and muscles.

Overall, weight-bearing exercises can be an effective way to promote bone health and reduce the risk of osteoporosis. These exercises can be performed on their own or as part of a broader exercise routine that includes other types of exercises such as resistance training, flexibility exercises, and balance and coordination exercises.

2. Resistance training

Resistance training involves exercises that use weights or resistance bands to build muscle strength. Examples include lifting weights, using resistance bands, and performing bodyweight exercises such as squats and lunges. Resistance training can also increase bone density by placing stress on the bones.

Resistance training can also help to improve muscle strength, which can in turn support the bones and reduce the risk of falls and fractures. Resistance exercises are particularly beneficial for individuals with osteoporosis, as they can help to maintain or improve bone density and promote bone remodeling. These exercises can be performed using weights, resistance bands, or even just bodyweight, and can target different muscle groups in the body. It's important to start with lighter weights and progress gradually to avoid injury and ensure proper form.

3. Balance and coordination exercises

Balance and coordination exercises focus on improving stability and body awareness, which can be especially helpful for individuals with osteoporosis who may be at increased risk of falls and fractures.

These exercises typically involve slow, controlled movements that challenge the body's balance and coordination. They can also help to improve posture and flexibility, which can further reduce the risk of falls.

Examples include yoga, tai chi, and Pilates.

4. Flexibility exercises

Flexibility exercises focus on stretching and lengthening the muscles, tendons, and ligaments around the joints, helping to improve joint mobility and range of motion thereby reducing the risk of injury.

Improved flexibility can also reduce the risk of falls and other injuries by allowing for better control and balance during physical activity.

Examples of flexibility exercises include yoga, Pilates, stretching exercises, and mobility drills.

5. High-impact exercises

High-impact exercises, such as jumping, can help to stimulate bone remodeling and increase bone density. However, individuals with osteoporosis should use caution when performing high-impact exercises, as they can increase the risk of fractures.

While high-impact exercises can be beneficial for bone health, they may not be suitable for individuals with severe osteoporosis or those who are at a high risk of fractures.

It's important to consult with a healthcare professional before starting any high-impact exercise routine.

Furthermore, it's important to note that individuals with osteoporosis should consult with their healthcare provider before starting an exercise program. They may need to modify certain exercises or avoid certain activities altogether to reduce the risk of injury. Additionally, it's important to start slowly and gradually increase the intensity and duration of exercise over time.

Specific Benefits of Exercise for Osteoporosis

Osteoporosis is a condition in which the bones become weak and brittle, increasing the risk of fractures. Exercise can play an important role in the management and prevention of osteoporosis, providing several specific benefits for individuals with this condition. Let's explore these benefits in detail:

1. Increased bone density

Weight-bearing and resistance exercises have been shown to stimulate bone remodeling and increase bone density. As bone density is a key indicator of bone strength, increasing it through exercise can help to strengthen the bones and reduce the risk of fractures.

This can help to strengthen the bones and reduce the risk of fractures. Weight-bearing exercises, such as walking, jogging, and stair climbing, involve placing weight on the bones and can stimulate the production of new bone tissue. Resistance exercises, such as weight lifting and bodyweight exercises, involve applying resistance to the bones and can help to maintain or improve bone density.

Weight-bearing exercises involve placing weight on the bones, which causes them to experience small amounts of stress. This stress stimulates the osteoblasts to produce new bone tissue, which increases bone density over time. Examples of weight-bearing exercises include walking, jogging, hiking, dancing, and stair climbing.

Resistance exercises, on the other hand, involve applying resistance to the bones, which also stimulates the osteoblasts to produce new bone tissue. Resistance exercises can include using weights, resistance bands, or bodyweight exercises such as push-ups, squats, and lunges. These exercises can help to maintain or improve bone density in individuals with osteoporosis.

It is important to note that the type, frequency, and intensity of exercise can all impact its effectiveness in increasing bone density. It is recommended that individuals with osteoporosis engage in weight-bearing and resistance exercises at least two to three times per week, with a focus on gradually increasing the intensity and weight used over time. It is also important to consult with a healthcare professional before beginning an exercise program, especially if an individual has a history of fractures or other bone-related health conditions.

2. Improved balance and coordination

Osteoporosis can increase the risk of falls, which can lead to fractures. Balance and coordination exercises can help to improve balance and reduce the risk of falls. Yoga and tai chi are examples of exercises that can help to improve balance and coordination. These exercises focus on slow, controlled movements and can help to improve body awareness and balance.

In addition to yoga and tai chi, other exercises that can improve balance and coordination include Pilates and specific balance training exercises. Pilates is a form of exercise that emphasizes core strength, body alignment, and control of movement. It can help to improve balance by targeting the muscles that support the spine and pelvis. Balance training exercises, such as standing on one leg or performing exercises on an unstable surface, can also help to improve balance and reduce the risk of falls.

Improving balance and coordination can also help to improve confidence and reduce the fear of falling, which can have a positive impact on daily activities and overall quality of life for individuals with osteoporosis.

3. Improved muscle strength

Resistance training can help to improve muscle strength, which can reduce the risk of falls and fractures. Strong muscles can help to support the bones and improve overall physical function. Resistance exercises can include weight lifting, bodyweight exercises, and resistance bands.

Additionally, weight-bearing exercises such as walking, jogging, and stair climbing can also help to improve muscle strength. When muscles contract against the resistance of body weight or external weights, they create tension on the bones that can stimulate the formation of new bone tissue. This process not only increases bone density but also strengthens the muscles, which in turn can help to prevent falls and fractures.

Moreover, as people age, they tend to lose muscle mass and strength, which can contribute to the development of osteoporosis. Exercise, particularly resistance training, can help to slow or even reverse this process by promoting the growth and maintenance of muscle tissue. This can have a positive impact on overall health and function, as well as reducing the risk of fractures.

4. Reduced risk of fracture

Regular exercise can help to reduce the risk of fractures by improving bone density, balance, and coordination. Regular exercise can help to reduce the risk of fractures in several ways.

First, exercise can improve bone density and strength, making bones less likely to break under stress. Second, exercise can improve balance, coordination, and muscle strength, which can reduce the risk of falls that can lead to fractures. Third, exercise can improve overall physical function, reducing the risk of injuries from accidents or other types of trauma.

Research has shown that exercise can be an effective way to reduce the risk of fractures in people with osteoporosis. A study published in the Journal of Bone and Mineral Research found that a year-long exercise program that included weight-bearing and resistance exercises reduced the risk of fractures in postmenopausal women with osteoporosis. Another study published in the same journal found that a 12-month exercise program that included resistance training and balance exercises reduced the risk of falls and fractures in women with osteoporosis.

Overall, regular exercise can be an important part of a comprehensive approach to managing osteoporosis and reducing the risk of fractures. It is important to work with a healthcare professional to develop an exercise program that is safe and effective for your individual needs and health status.

5. Improved joint mobility

Osteoporosis can cause stiffness and reduced mobility in the joints. Flexibility exercises, such as stretching and yoga, can help to improve joint mobility and reduce the risk of injury. These exercises can help to improve range of motion and reduce stiffness in the joints.

To further elaborate on the point, exercise can help to improve joint mobility, which is especially important for people with osteoporosis who may experience joint stiffness and reduced mobility. Flexibility exercises, such as stretching and yoga, can help to improve joint mobility and range of motion. Stretching can help to loosen tight muscles and increase flexibility, while yoga can help to improve balance, coordination, and overall physical function.

In addition, low-impact exercises such as swimming and cycling can also help to improve joint mobility without putting excessive strain on the joints. These exercises can help to reduce stiffness and increase mobility in the joints, while also providing cardiovascular benefits.

Improved joint mobility can also have indirect benefits for bone health. For example, improved joint mobility can allow for a wider range of movement during exercise, which can help to stimulate bone remodeling and increase bone density. Additionally, improved joint mobility can help to reduce the risk of falls and other injuries, which can in turn reduce the risk of fracture

6. Improved overall health

Exercise can provide several other health benefits that can improve overall quality of life for individuals with osteoporosis. Regular exercise can provide a range of health benefits beyond just improving bone health for individuals with osteoporosis. Here are a few additional benefits:

7. Improved cardiovascular health

Regular exercise can help to strengthen the heart and improve cardiovascular health. This can reduce the risk of heart disease, stroke, and other cardiovascular problems, which are more common in individuals with osteoporosis.

8. Reduced risk of chronic diseases

Exercise has been shown to reduce the risk of chronic diseases such as type 2 diabetes, obesity, and certain types of cancer. These conditions are also associated with an increased risk of osteoporosis, so reducing the risk of these diseases can help to prevent osteoporosis.

9. Improved mood and mental health

Exercise has been shown to improve mood and reduce symptoms of anxiety and depression. Individuals with osteoporosis may be at an increased risk of depression and anxiety due to the impact of the disease on their daily activities, so exercise can be an effective way to improve mental health.

10. Increased overall physical function

Exercise can improve overall physical function, which can help individuals with osteoporosis maintain their independence and quality of life. Improving strength, flexibility, balance, and coordination can help individuals with osteoporosis perform daily activities with greater ease and confidence.

Overall, regular exercise can provide a range of benefits for individuals with osteoporosis beyond just improving bone health. It is important to consult with a healthcare professional before starting any exercise program, especially if you have osteoporosis or any other medical conditions.

11. Increase Bone density

Bone density is an important measure of bone health, and exercise has been shown to increase it in individuals with osteoporosis. Bone density is a measure of the amount of mineral in bone tissue, and it is often used as an indicator of bone strength. The higher the bone density, the stronger the bone.

When an individual engages in weight-bearing or resistance exercise, the bones experience small amounts of stress. This stress stimulates the osteoblasts (cells that produce new bone tissue) to produce new bone tissue, which increases bone density over time. This effect is particularly pronounced in individuals with osteoporosis, as their bones may have experienced significant mineral loss.

By increasing bone density through exercise, individuals with osteoporosis can improve their bone quality and reduce their risk of fractures. This is especially important for individuals with osteoporosis, as they are at an increased risk of fractures due to weakened bone structure.

It's important to note that the specific benefits of exercise for osteoporosis may vary depending on the individual's age, overall health, and the type and intensity of exercise performed. It's important for individuals with osteoporosis to work with their healthcare provider and a qualified exercise professional to develop a safe and effective exercise program that meets their individual needs and goals.

Chapter Six

Designing an Exercise Program for Osteoporosis

Designing an exercise program for osteoporosis should be done in consultation with a healthcare professional, such as a doctor or physical therapist, to ensure safety and effectiveness. The program should include a combination of weight-bearing, resistance, balance, coordination, and flexibility exercises.

Here are some general guidelines for designing an exercise program for osteoporosis:

1. **Start slowly**

If you are new to exercise or have been inactive for a while, start slowly and gradually increase the intensity and duration of your workouts over time.

2. Include a variety of exercises

A combination of weight-bearing, resistance, balance, coordination, and flexibility exercises can provide the most benefits for individuals with osteoporosis.

3. Choose exercises that are safe for you

Some high-impact exercises, such as jumping or running, may not be safe for individuals with osteoporosis. Consult with a healthcare professional to determine which exercises are safe for you.

4. Use proper form

Using proper form when performing exercises is essential for safety and effectiveness. Consider working with a certified personal trainer or physical therapist to learn proper form.

5. Progress gradually

As your strength and fitness improve, gradually increase the intensity and duration of your workouts. But avoid overdoing it and causing injury.

6. Allow for rest and recovery

Rest and recovery are important for preventing injury and allowing the body to adapt to the stresses of exercise. Aim for at least one rest day per week.

7. Stay consistent

Consistency is key for seeing results from exercise. Aim for at least 30 minutes of moderate-intensity exercise on most days of the week.

Remember to consult with a healthcare professional before starting any new exercise program, especially if you have osteoporosis or other medical conditions.

Factors to consider when designing an exercise program

When designing an exercise program for osteoporosis, there are several factors to consider. These include:

1. Medical history

It's important to consider any past or present medical conditions that may impact the safety and effectiveness of exercise.

2. Fitness level

The current fitness level of the individual should be considered when developing an exercise program. This will help to determine the appropriate intensity and type of exercises.

3. Bone density

The individual's bone density should be evaluated to determine the appropriate exercises to promote bone health without risking fractures.

4. Age and gender

Age and gender can impact the risk of osteoporosis and the effectiveness of exercise interventions.

5. Personal preferences

The individual's personal preferences and interests should also be considered when designing an exercise program, as this can improve adherence and overall success.

6. Availability of resources

The availability of resources, such as equipment or facilities, should also be considered when designing an exercise program.

7. Potential contraindications

Certain exercises may be contraindicated for individuals with certain conditions or injuries, so it's important to consider potential contraindications when developing an exercise program.

General guidelines for exercise with osteoporosis

Here are some general guidelines for exercise with osteoporosis:

1. Consult with your healthcare provider before starting any exercise program.
2. Choose exercises that are appropriate for your fitness level and physical abilities.
3. Incorporate weight-bearing and resistance exercises to help improve bone density and reduce the risk of fractures.
4. Include exercises that focus on balance and coordination to reduce the risk of falls.
5. Gradually increase the intensity and duration of exercise over time, but avoid overexertion or excessive impact.
6. Allow for adequate rest and recovery between exercise sessions.

7. Consider working with a certified personal trainer or physical therapist who has experience working with individuals with osteoporosis to develop a safe and effective exercise program.
8. Be consistent with your exercise routine, aiming for at least 30 minutes of moderate-intensity exercise most days of the week.
9. Stay hydrated and properly fuel your body with a balanced diet to support your exercise program and overall health.
10. Wear appropriate footwear and clothing for your exercise routine to ensure proper support and reduce the risk of injury.
11. Avoid exercises or activities that may put excessive stress on the spine or increase the risk of falls, such as high-impact exercises or exercises that involve bending forward at the waist.
12. Be mindful of any pain or discomfort during exercise and modify or stop exercises as needed.
13. Consider incorporating a variety of exercises to prevent boredom and maintain motivation.
14. Monitor your progress and adjust your exercise program as needed to continue challenging your body and achieving your goals.
15. Remember that consistency is key to achieving the benefits of exercise for osteoporosis. Stick to your routine and be patient with the results, as improvements in bone density and overall health may take time to see.

Examples of exercise routines for osteoporosis

Here are some examples of exercise routines for individuals with osteoporosis:

1. Beginner Routine

Warm-up

5-10 minutes of walking or marching in place.

Strength Training

2 sets of 8-12 reps of bodyweight exercises such as squats, lunges, push-ups, and wall sits.

Balance Training

5-10 minutes of exercises such as standing on one leg, heel-to-toe walk, and side leg lifts.

Cool-down

5-10 minutes of stretching exercises such as hamstring stretches, quad stretches, and calf stretches.

2. Intermediate Routine

Warm-up

5-10 minutes of low-impact cardio exercises such as walking or stationary cycling.

Strength Training

3 sets of 8-12 reps of resistance exercises such as dumbbell squats, lunges, bicep curls, tricep extensions, and chest presses.

Balance Training

10-15 minutes of exercises such as yoga, tai chi, or Pilates.

Cool-down

5-10 minutes of stretching exercises such as hip flexor stretches, shoulder stretches, and back stretches.

3. Advanced Routine

Warm-up

10-15 minutes of low-impact cardio exercises such as jogging, jumping jacks, or rowing machine.

Strength Training

3-4 sets of 8-12 reps of resistance exercises such as barbell squats, deadlifts, bench presses, and pull-ups.

Balance Training

15-20 minutes of exercises such as single-leg balance, Bosu ball exercises, or stability ball exercises.

Cool-down

5-10 minutes of stretching exercises such as full body stretches and foam rolling.

Remember to adjust the intensity and duration of exercises based on your fitness level and physical abilities, and to always consult with your healthcare provider before starting a new exercise routine.

Chapter Seven

Possible risks and side effects of exercise with osteoporosis

Osteoporosis is a medical condition that weakens bones, making them fragile and more prone to fractures. While exercise is generally recommended for people with osteoporosis, there are some possible risks and side effects that you should be aware of:

1. Fractures

If you have severe osteoporosis, certain high-impact exercises can increase your risk of fractures. For example, exercises like jumping, running, or high-impact aerobics can put too much stress on your bones and increase your risk of fractures.

High-impact exercises can be risky for people with severe osteoporosis because their bones are more fragile and prone to fractures. When you perform high-impact exercises, such as running or jumping, the impact of your feet hitting the ground can put significant stress on your bones, which may cause fractures or other injuries.

This is why it's important to consult with your doctor or a physical therapist to develop a safe and appropriate exercise program that takes into account your individual needs and level of bone density. They may recommend low-impact exercises, such as walking, cycling, or swimming that provide the benefits of exercise without the risk of fractures. Additionally, it's important to wear appropriate footwear and use proper technique during exercise to minimize the risk of injury.

2. Muscle and joint pain

If you have osteoporosis, you may experience muscle and joint pain during or after exercise. This may be due to weakened bones, which can cause additional stress on your muscles and joints.

People with osteoporosis may experience muscle and joint pain during or after exercise due to the weakened bones. Weakened bones can put extra stress on the muscles and joints, making them work harder to support the body during exercise. This can lead to muscle and joint pain or discomfort.

However, it's important to note that exercise can also help strengthen the muscles and improve joint flexibility, which may ultimately reduce pain and improve mobility. If you experience muscle or joint pain during or after exercise, it's important to talk to your doctor or physical therapist. They can help you modify your exercise routine or recommend stretches or other exercises that can help alleviate pain and discomfort.

Additionally, it's important to warm up properly before exercise and stretch afterward to prevent muscle soreness and injury.

3. Loss of balance

Osteoporosis can increase the risk of falls and loss of balance, which can lead to fractures or other injuries. When the bones are weakened due to osteoporosis, they may be less able to support the body's weight and maintain balance during exercise. Certain exercises, such as those that involve standing on one foot, or those that require quick changes in direction, can be particularly challenging for people with osteoporosis and increase the risk of falls.

However, balance exercises can also be beneficial in improving balance and reducing the risk of falls. It's important to consult with your doctor or physical therapist to develop a safe and appropriate exercise program that takes into account your individual needs and level of bone density. They may recommend exercises that improve balance and coordination, such as yoga or tai chi, or provide guidance on how to modify exercises to reduce the risk of falls.

Additionally, it's important to exercise in a safe and well-lit environment, wear appropriate footwear, and use assistive devices as needed to prevent falls.

4. Spinal compression fractures

Certain exercises that involve bending forward or twisting the spine such as sit-ups, crunches, can increase the risk of spinal compression fractures in people with osteoporosis as these types of fractures can cause severe pain and may require medical attention.

Spinal compression fractures occur when the vertebrae in the spine collapse or become compressed, which can cause severe pain, limited mobility, and other complications. Exercises that involve excessive bending, twisting, or sudden movements can put additional stress on the spine and increase the risk of these types of fractures.

To reduce the risk of spinal compression fractures, it's important to avoid exercises that involve excessive bending or twisting of the spine, such as sit-ups, crunches, or exercises that involve twisting motions. Your doctor or physical therapist can recommend exercises that strengthen the core and improve posture without putting too much stress on the spine.

Additionally, it's important to use proper form during exercise and to avoid jerky or sudden movements that can increase the risk of injury. If you experience back pain or other symptoms after exercise, it's important to consult with your doctor to rule out the possibility of a spinal compression fracture or other injury.

5. Overexertion

People with osteoporosis may also be at risk of overexertion during exercise. Overexertion during exercise can put additional stress on the bones and muscles, which can increase the risk of injury and exacerbate symptoms of osteoporosis. It can lead to fatigue, weakness, and injury. It is important to start slowly and gradually increase the intensity of your exercise routine to avoid overexertion.

People with osteoporosis may be more susceptible to overexertion due to reduced bone density, muscle weakness, or other factors. To reduce the risk of overexertion, it's important to start slowly and gradually increase the intensity of your exercise routine over time.

Your doctor or physical therapist can help you develop an exercise program that is tailored to your individual needs and level of bone density. They may recommend exercises that are low-impact and less likely to cause injury, such as walking, swimming, or cycling.

Additionally, it's important to listen to your body and take breaks as needed during exercise. If you experience pain, weakness, or other symptoms during exercise, it's important to stop and rest or seek medical attention if necessary.

6. Spinal deformity

People with advanced osteoporosis may be at risk of developing a spinal deformity called kyphosis, which is a forward curvature of the upper spine that can cause back pain, difficulty breathing, and poor posture.

Certain exercises that involve twisting or bending the spine may worsen kyphosis and increase the risk of spinal compression fractures. To reduce the risk of kyphosis and other spinal deformities, it's important to maintain good posture and avoid exercises that put excessive stress on the spine.

Your doctor or physical therapist can recommend exercises that strengthen the back muscles and improve posture without exacerbating kyphosis.

Additionally, it's important to use proper form during exercise and avoid jerky or sudden movements that can increase the risk of injury. If you experience back pain or other symptoms during exercise, it's important to consult with your doctor to rule out the possibility of a spinal compression fracture or other injury.

7. Fractures from falls

People with osteoporosis are at an increased risk of fractures from falls. It's important to take precautions to prevent falls, such as wearing appropriate footwear with good grip, using assistive devices like canes or walkers if needed and making sure your home is free of hazards such as loose rugs or electrical cords.

Falling can cause serious injuries, especially for people with weakened bones.

You can also improve your balance and coordination with exercises that focus on these areas. Your doctor or physical therapist can recommend exercises and strategies to reduce the risk of falls and fractures. Additionally, if you experience dizziness or balance problems, it's important to discuss this with your doctor as they may be able to help identify underlying causes and recommend appropriate treatments.

8. Decreased bone density

While exercise can help improve bone density, certain types of exercise, such as low-impact exercises like swimming or cycling do not provide as much stress on the bones and may not be as effective at improving bone density or promote bone growth. It's important to include weight-bearing exercises in your routine.

Weight-bearing exercises, such as walking, jogging, or lifting weights, can help stimulate bone growth and improve bone density. These exercises put stress on the bones, which can help them become stronger. However, it's important to note that any type of exercise is better than no exercise, and low-impact exercises like swimming can still provide many other health benefits, such as improved cardiovascular health and muscle strength. It's important to talk to your doctor or a physical therapist to determine the best types of exercise for your individual needs and health status.

To reduce the risk of these side effects, it's important to consult with your doctor before starting any exercise program. Your doctor may recommend exercises that are low-impact, such as swimming, walking, or yoga, which can help strengthen your bones and improve your balance without putting too much stress on your body. Additionally, it's important to wear appropriate footwear and protective gear, such as helmets or wrist guards, during exercise to prevent injuries.

Chapter Eight

Prevention of Osteoporosis

Osteoporosis is a "silent" illness because it frequently causes no symptoms, and you might not even be aware that you have it until you break a bone. In elderly men and postmenopausal women, osteoporosis is the leading cause of fractures. Any bone can break, but the hip, wrist, and vertebrae in the spine are the most commonly affected.

Prevention of osteoporosis involves lifestyle modifications and sometimes medical interventions. You can take a number of steps as an adult to support the preservation of strong bones and prevent untimely bone thinning.

Simple dietary adjustments, regular exercise, and a change in bad lifestyle choices will not only help you prevent osteoporosis but also improve your overall health.

Here are some ways to prevent osteoporosis:

1. **Adequate calcium and vitamin D intake**

Calcium and vitamin D are essential for strong bones. It is recommended that adults consume 1,000-1,200 mg of calcium and 800-1,000 IU of vitamin D per day. Good sources of calcium include dairy products, leafy greens, and fortified foods. Vitamin D can be obtained through sun exposure or from supplements.

2. Regular exercise

Weight-bearing exercises, such as walking, jogging, and weightlifting, can help to build and maintain bone density. Aim for at least 30 minutes of exercise most days of the week.

3. Avoid smoking and excessive alcohol consumption

Smoking and excessive alcohol consumption can lead to decreased bone density and an increased risk of fractures. Quitting smoking and limiting alcohol intake can help to prevent osteoporosis.

4. Medical interventions

For individuals at high risk of osteoporosis, medical interventions may be necessary. These may include medications such as bisphosphonates or hormone replacement therapy (HRT), which can help to slow bone loss and reduce fracture risk.

5. Fall prevention

Falls are the cause of fractures in individuals with osteoporosis. Taking steps to prevent falls, such as removing tripping hazards from the home and using assistive devices like canes or walkers, can help to prevent fractures.

6. Regular bone density testing

Individuals at high risk of osteoporosis may benefit from regular bone density testing to monitor changes in bone density and evaluate the effectiveness of interventions.

7. Healthy diet

A healthy diet that is rich in fruits, vegetables, whole grains, and lean proteins can help to promote overall health and prevent osteoporosis. Consuming foods that are high in calcium and vitamin D, such as milk, yogurt, cheese, and fatty fish, can also help to improve bone health.

8. Avoid certain medications

Certain medications, such as glucocorticoids and some anticonvulsants, can increase the risk of osteoporosis. Individuals taking these medications should talk to their healthcare provider about the potential risks and benefits and explore alternative treatment options if necessary.

9. Hormone replacement therapy

Hormone replacement therapy (HRT) may be an option for women who have gone through menopause and are at high risk of osteoporosis. HRT can help to increase estrogen levels, which can slow bone loss and reduce fracture risk. However, HRT is not appropriate for all women, and the risks and benefits should be carefully considered before starting treatment.

10. Manage medical conditions

Certain medical conditions, such as hyperthyroidism, inflammatory bowel disease, and celiac disease, can increase the risk of osteoporosis. Managing these conditions and working with a healthcare provider to monitor bone health can help to prevent osteoporosis.

11. Maintain a healthy weight

Being underweight or overweight can increase the risk of osteoporosis. Maintaining a healthy weight through a balanced diet and regular exercise can help to prevent osteoporosis.

12. Consider supplements

In addition to getting nutrients through diet, supplements such as calcium, vitamin D, and magnesium can help to improve bone health. However, it is important to talk to a healthcare provider before starting any new supplements to ensure that they are safe and effective.

It is important to note that while supplements can be helpful, it is generally recommended to get nutrients through a balanced diet whenever possible. Additionally, taking high doses of certain supplements, such as calcium, can have negative health effects, so it is important to follow recommended dosages and consult with a healthcare provider.

Chapter Nine

Nutrition for Osteoporosis

Nutrition plays a critical role in managing osteoporosis. A balanced and nutrient-rich diet can help slow down bone loss, maintain bone strength, and prevent fractures. Here are some key nutrients to focus on:

1. Calcium

Calcium is essential for building and maintaining strong bones. Good sources of calcium include dairy products, leafy green vegetables, and fortified foods such as cereals and juices.

Adequate calcium intake is important for bone health, and it's recommended that adults aim for 1000-1200 mg of calcium per day.

Good sources of calcium include:

- Dairy products, such as milk, yogurt, and cheese.
- Leafy green vegetables, such as kale, collard greens, and spinach.
- Fortified foods, such as cereals, bread, and orange juice.
- Tofu

- Canned fish with bones, such as salmon and sardines.

It's important to note that calcium supplements may be necessary for some people to reach their recommended daily intake. However, it's generally recommended to get most of your calcium from food sources rather than supplements.

2. Vitamin D

Vitamin D helps the body absorb calcium and promote bone growth. The primary source of vitamin D is sunlight, but it can also be found in fatty fish, egg yolks, and fortified foods.

Vitamin D plays a crucial role in calcium absorption and bone health. The body can produce vitamin D with the help of sunlight, but it can also be obtained through dietary sources such as fatty fish (e.g. salmon, tuna, and mackerel), egg yolks, and fortified foods like milk, cereal, and orange juice.

In some cases, a vitamin D supplement may be recommended by a doctor or registered dietitian to ensure adequate intake.

3. Magnesium

Magnesium is also important for bone health, as it helps the body absorb and use calcium. Good sources of magnesium include nuts, seeds, whole grains, and leafy green vegetables.

Magnesium is a mineral that works closely with calcium and vitamin D to maintain strong bones. It plays a crucial role in bone formation and helps the body absorb calcium from the diet.

In addition to the sources you mentioned, other good sources of magnesium include legumes, avocados, bananas, and dark chocolate.

4. Protein

Adequate protein intake is essential for maintaining muscle mass and bone strength. Good sources of protein include lean meats, poultry, fish, beans, and dairy products.

Protein is important for bone health because it helps with the absorption of calcium and promotes bone growth. It's also important for maintaining muscle mass, which is essential for balance and reducing the risk of falls.

It's recommended to aim for a balanced intake of protein from both animal and plant sources.

5. Vitamin K

Vitamin K helps regulate calcium in the body and promotes bone health. Vitamin K plays an important role in bone health by helping to activate a protein called osteocalcin, which is involved in bone formation.

Good sources of vitamin K include dark leafy greens, such as spinach, kale, and collard greens, as well as broccoli, Brussels sprouts, and green beans.

6. Phosphorus

Phosphorus works with calcium to build strong bones. Phosphorus is an essential mineral that works with calcium to build and maintain strong bones. It plays a vital role in bone mineralization, which is the process by which calcium and other minerals are deposited in bones, making them hard and strong.

Good sources of phosphorus include dairy products, meat, fish, and poultry. It's important to consume phosphorus in balance with calcium intake, as an excessive amount of phosphorus can interfere with calcium absorption and lead to weakened bones.

Consequently, in addition to these nutrients, it's important to limit intake of foods and drinks that can weaken bones, such as alcohol and caffeine. It's also important to maintain a healthy body weight, as being underweight can increase the risk of osteoporosis. It's recommended to talk to a doctor or registered dietitian for personalized nutrition recommendations to manage osteoporosis.

Conclusion

Osteoporosis is a condition characterized by weak and brittle bones, which increases the risk of fractures. Regular exercise can help improve bone density and reduce the risk of falls and fractures. Weight-bearing exercises, such as walking, jogging, and strength training, are particularly beneficial for building strong bones.

However, certain types of exercise, such as those that involve bending or twisting the spine, may increase the risk of spinal fractures. A balanced and nutrient-rich diet is also important for managing osteoporosis, with a focus on calcium, vitamin D, magnesium, protein, vitamin K, and phosphorus.

It is important to seek guidance from healthcare professionals, such as a doctor, physical therapist, or certified exercise specialist, before starting an exercise program for osteoporosis. They can help create a safe and effective exercise plan that is tailored to your individual needs and fitness level.

They can also provide guidance on how to perform exercises correctly, monitor progress, and make adjustments to the program as needed. This can help prevent injuries and maximize the benefits of exercise   for   osteoporosis.

REFERRENCES

https://www.niams.nih.gov/health-topics/osteoporosis#

https://www.osteoporosis.foundation/patients/prevention